I0428496

HIIT Training Program

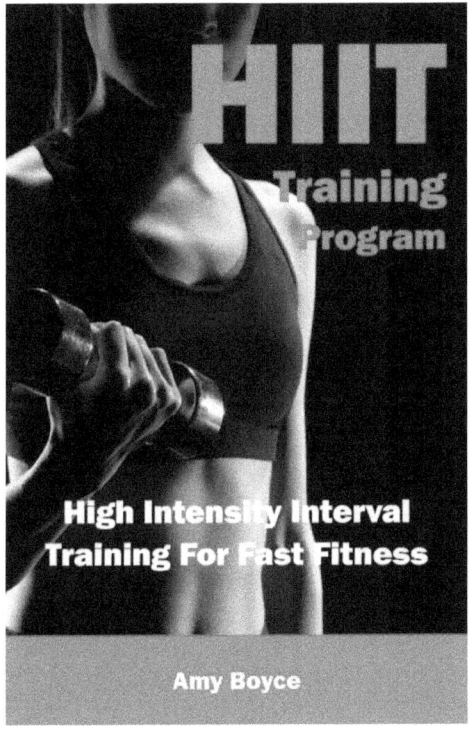

High Intensity Interval Training for Fast Fitness

HIIT Training Program:
High Intensity Interval Training for Fast Fitness
by **Amy Boyce**

Printed in the United States of America

Health Disclaimer

All material in this report is provided for your information only and may not be construed as medical advice or instruction. No action or inaction should be taken based solely on the contents of this information; instead, readers should consult appropriate health professionals on any matter relating to their health and well-being.

The information and opinions expressed here are believed to be accurate, based on the best judgment available to the authors, and readers who fail to consult with appropriate health authorities assume the risk of any injuries.

Table of Contents

HIIT Training Program

Introduction

HIIT Training Program

One of the problems with exercise is that it can take a long time to get the results you're looking for. High intensity interval training (HIIT) is one of the most effective methods of exercise. It is now the top workout for many professional athletes who need to get fit fast. In this guide, you'll learn how you can gain massive fitness results without spending hours at the gym.

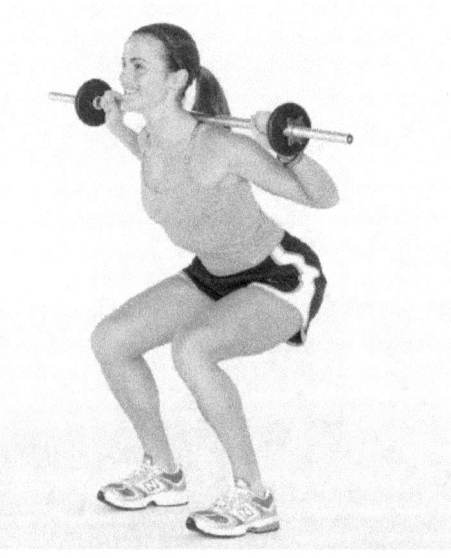

We all realize the importance of regular exercise, not only for the overall health benefits, but also to gain energy, lose weight and gain strength. The

HIIT Training Program

problem is, if we have to invest a lot of money or time on equipment gym memberships, or coaching, it can be easy to not make exercise a priority.

One of the most powerful things about HIIT is that it really fits into our busy lifestyle and, in many cases, we can do it at home with some basic equipment. This is one workout method that does not need a lot of fancy equipment or massive amounts of time to see results.

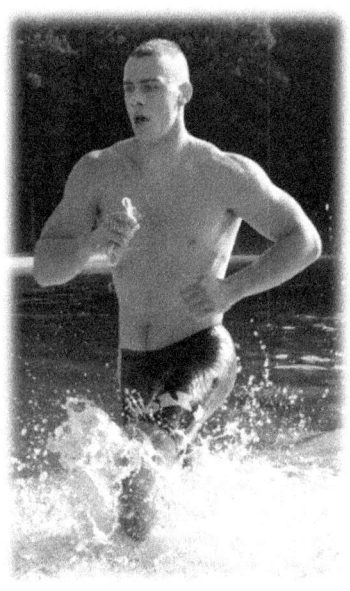

HIIT Training Program

The basic premise of HIIT is to engage small intervals of exercise that is of high intensity. In between, moderate or low levels of exertion are being used. By alternating between very hard, but brief, exercise duration, and then a less intense one, the metabolism keeps working in the heart rate stays up long after the session is finished. What's great about HI IT is that you are building strength and also improving your endurance levels.

This guide covers everything you need to get started with an effective HIIT program. You'll learn the benefits, how to get started, and how to effectively work out.

Chapter 1

The Many Benefits of HIIT

HIIT Training Program

HIIT has really surged in popularity the last few years. The main reason is because of its effectiveness. This is the best workout going for burning fat, building muscle and overall toning. And, there is no need to spending hours at the gym. In addition, HIIT encompasses many different exercises so there is no room for boredom.

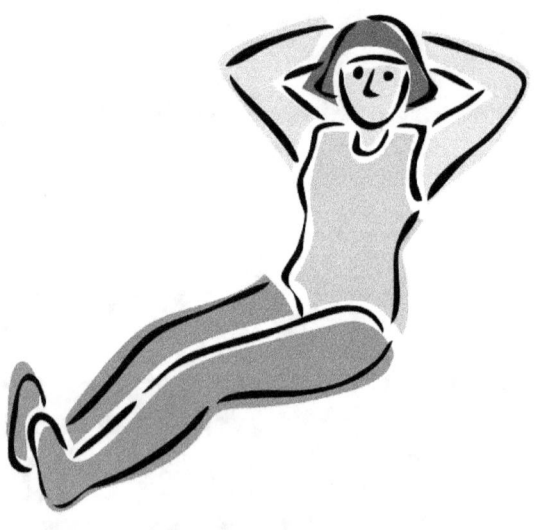

HIIT Training Program

Here are a few more benefits and reasons why you want to use HIIT to get the results you desire.

- Kick start your metabolism- this type of workout really boosts your metabolism and you'll still be burning fat after your workout for up to two days.

- Get both anaerobic and aerobic benefits- one of the unique aspects of H IIT is that it both provides a cardio workout, and it also allows you to build lean muscle. This is a powerful combination.

- Easy and quick- most of the workouts can be done nearly anywhere, and are under 30 minutes in length. That means there are little to no excuses for getting a highly effective workout in.

- Reduce cardiovascular risks- intense activity with HIIT has been shown to lower the risks associated with different cardiovascular diseases.

HIIT Training Program

One of the main tenants of HIIT is the fact that the workout routine changes quickly. Not only will you be changing your pace throughout the workout, but there are many different methods you can use. This means your body does not get used to the exercise, and it also means you can get a full body workout very quickly. Like a professional athlete, you'll be able to get massive results in the least amount of time.

There are tons of myths and misconceptions about most exercise routines, but perhaps the worst are reserved for HIIT. Some people have hesitated starting this routine because they are confused about what the routine does, it's many benefits and the overall difficulty.

HIIT Training Program

Myths and misconceptions about HIIT

These are the six most common myths and misconceptions about the popular HIIT philosophy:

1. Only consistently hard cardio workouts burn fat. It's true that cardio does burn some fat, but it's not nearly as much as switching up the intensity or using weight. Experts have found that alternating the intensity, such as with HIIT, builds more muscle and burns additional fat.

2. A lower intensity workout for a long time is the key to burning fat. Most studies have found that the opposite is true and that you burn the most fat when working for intense, brief periods. HIIT combines both anaerobic and aerobic exercises so that you create a staggered interval routine that produces much better results in a shorter amount of time.

3. Diet doesn't matter if you exercise every day. This is completely false. There's no

way to get the dream body you always wanted if you constantly eating candy and fattening foods. If you really want to lose weight, then it's best to make healthy food choices each and every day, regardless of how much you exercise.

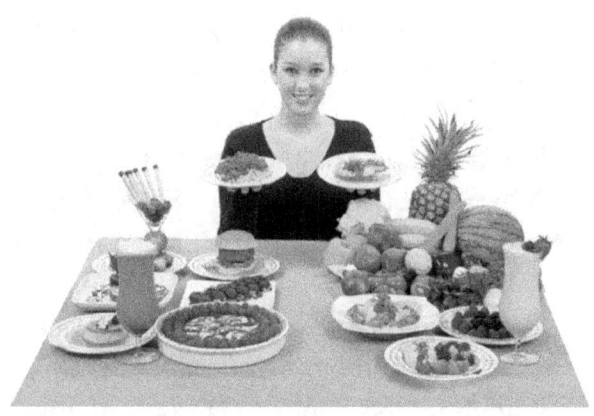

4. You'll lose weight and get fit by just doing your favorite exercise. If you want to achieve fast results and get really fit, then you need to add variety to your exercise routine. Rather than just walking or jogging, use other workouts like push-ups or weight training. This will also keep you from hitting a plateau.

HIIT Training Program

5. Working out in the morning is best for your metabolism because it ramps it up throughout the day. It's actually best to exercise when you can, rather than sticking to a specific time or hour. However, the one exception to this is if you have high blood pressure. You should then workout during the morning because studies have found that exercise reduces blood pressure for many hours.

6. There's an age bracket, and you're just too old. This is probably the worst misconception about HIIT and fitness in general. Anyone, of any age, can see real benefits from working out. The elderly will actually reduce their risk of bone and muscle disease while also improving their activity and quality of life.

If you're not working out or aren't getting the results you need, then remember that HIIT is a great way to get yourself started. If you have any doubts, then consult your physician to see which exercise is best for you.

HIIT Training Program

The Beginnings of HIIT

HIIT arose out of a number of academic and athletic-based research and studies. For example, Peter Coe developed a running regimen in the 1970s. He would have short runs of 200 meters followed by a short recovery before the next run started.

Fast forwarding to the beginning of the 2010s, Professor Izumi Tabata developed a program that was used to train Olympic skaters. Variations of the Tabata workout are still being used today, and are an essential component of HIIT training.

HIIT Training Program

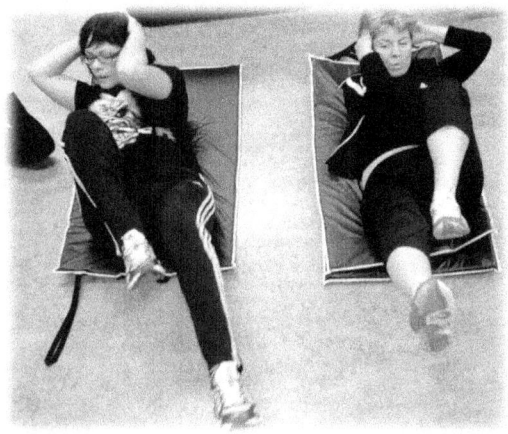

Another workout regimen originated by Prof. Martin Gibala in Canada was designed for less active people who have been inactive for a longer period of time. This included a short period of muscle warm-up, followed by high-intensity activity of 60 seconds duration, and 10 repetitions each high-intensity bursts was followed by 60 seconds of recovery and a five-minute cool down at the end of the session.

Jamie Timmons, a biology professor developed a workout that consists of an exercise bike pedaling for two minutes fast cycling at 20 seconds after each two-minute interval. This was recommended, along with a warm-up and cool down, to be

HIIT Training Program

performed three times a week for a three minute duration.

As you can see from these examples, HIIT training evolved from research and study of best practices for top-level athletes. It has been proven effective, and it is not some fly-by-night type of training.

HIIT Training Program

HIIT Effects on The Body

HIIT uses the principles of aerobic exercise to burn fat and build muscle. With aerobic exercise, your body needs more oxygen and that causes you to breathe deeper and faster so your body can receive more. The thing is, your muscles do burn and you have to make up for the oxygen use after you've exercise.

With each H IIT, you can give your body more time to recover. By working for shorter intervals and then having a lower intensity duration. This is actually easier on your body and provides more benefits. In addition, HIIT combines both the aerobic exercises and the anaerobic or strength building exercises. This allows you to burn fat and increase muscle more efficiently.

Getting Started With HIIT

You'll want to evaluate your level of fitness before you get started within HIIT training program. For example, if you have been inactive for a long period of time or are massively overweight, you should definitely consult your doctor before you start any type of exercise program.

In addition, because of the high intensity level of HIIIT, you will want to prepare your body before you get started. A good way to get started is to walk daily for 30 minutes at least for 30 days. Yoga is also a great place to build in some strength and increase balance.

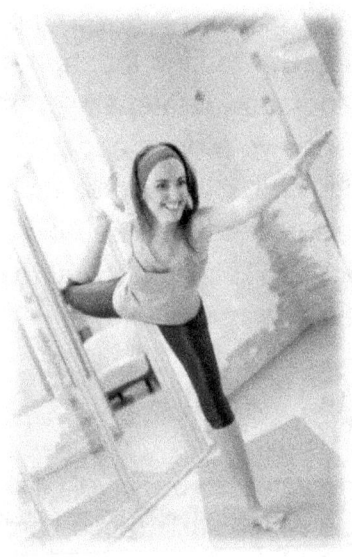

HIIT Training Program

Here are some specific guidelines to follow for this exercise program:

- Build up gradually with your HIIT exercises, and don't do the highest intensity right away.

- Make sure you warm-up before your workout and cool down after each workout.

- This program is for those who want to lose fat without losing muscle, and also increase their cardio and endurance levels of fitness.

- Make sure you can exercise for 20 to 30 minutes at about 75% of your highest effort before you start and HIIT program.

- Make sure you are giving it your full effort during the high level part of the interval. When your muscles start burning, you're now in the anaerobic zone and you should slow down and moved to the lower intensity interval at that point.

HIIT Training Program

- Your heart rate should drop to around 70% during your recovery interval, if you are finding that is not happening, add more time to your recovery or decrease the time for the work interval.

- When you first start, your recovery will last up to four minutes. Over time, this can be decreased if you're high intensity sections are shorter.

- If you have trouble breathing or experience any other type of difficulties during your workout, don't just stop. Instead, begin your cool down section.

This is going to be an intense workout, so it is important that you get an approval from your doctor or healthcare professional before you start. However, if you are seriously out of shape as I mentioned previously, you should get your strength and stamina up by walking or doing another form of exercise for at least 30 days before you start HIIT. Another way you can ensure the safety of your workout is to stay hydrated before and after your workout.

HIIT Training Program

HIIT Framework

Your overall workout will consists of a 5 to 10 minute warm-up. Then, you will start your high level intensity for an average of one minute. Next, you will recover at a lower level for 2 to 3 minutes, and then repeat the high-intensity again. You can start with just a few intervals, which are the sections of high followed by low or no intensity, and see if you can increase of over time to more cycles, such as 10 to 12.

In the next chapter, I'll discuss how you can get started and what to do to move to more advanced workout levels over time.

Chapter 2

Starting Out and Moving Up with Your HIIT Workouts

HIIT Training Program

In this chapter, I'll go over the different levels of activity, so you will know where to get started and when you can move to the next level. If you're not sure which your fitness level is, start with the beginners level and then move up as needed. If you've already been working out for a while and have a high level of fitness, you can get started at the intermediate or perhaps even the advanced level.

Once you've been doing this for a bit, and you want more of a challenge, feel free to move to the next level. If that proves to be too difficult, you can always go back to the beginner, but you can increase your workout by increasing the number of cycles you do. Because of this flexibility, it is easy to keep up a challenging workout, no matter where you are.

Getting Started at the Beginner Level

It's exciting to get started with this as a beginner, because you'll see that you'll be able to tone, lose weight, and gain muscle in a shorter amount of time that you would with other workouts.

HIIT Training Program

Here are some tips to get started with HIIT:

- When you're just getting started , aim to do it 2 to 3 times a week, because of its intensity, you don't need to do it more than that.

- Start with very small intervals of high-intensity activity. After the warm-up, you can start with as little as 20 seconds of intensity, followed by 40 seconds at a slower pace. Do this interval cycle for about 15 minutes and then cool down for five minutes.

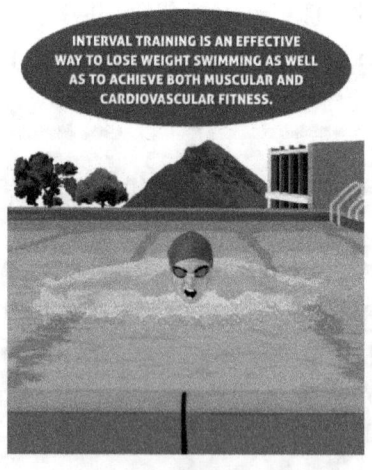

INTERVAL TRAINING IS AN EFFECTIVE WAY TO LOSE WEIGHT SWIMMING AS WELL AS TO ACHIEVE BOTH MUSCULAR AND CARDIOVASCULAR FITNESS.

HIIT Training Program

- Start with a cardio exercise you already like. For example, you can do cycling, swimming, running, or even dancing. Change it up over time to provide your body with the challenge.

- Over time, decrease your resting time. After two weeks, decrease your lower activity or rest intervals by about 10 seconds. After about a month, you can then try increasing your high-intensity interval by 10 seconds. Many people use a timer. They can set that will beep at each interval, so they don't have to look at the clock during their workout.

- Listen to your body. If the intensity is too much, you can always lower the amount of time for your intensity interval, and increase the amount of time for your rest interval.

Moving To the Next HIIT Level

After anywhere from six weeks to two months, you may be ready to increase your intensity level and

HIIT Training Program

start more intermediate level training. The main difference is making your intensity level higher, and decreasing your rest time. For example, you may do a high-intensity jump rope workout for 40 seconds, followed by the 22nd rest period. You would then cycle through this anywhere from 10 to 20 times.

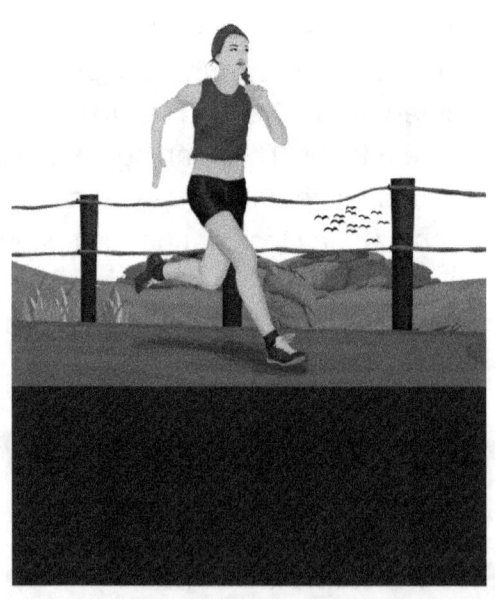

Jogging or running also lends itself to the intermediate levels. For example, you could run

HIIT Training Program

fast for one minute, and then slow to a jog for one minute. Alternate between 10 to 15 minutes. This is a great workout and will help you get fit very quickly.

Advanced Levels of HIIT

This is the levels where Olympic athletes use to train with. This is where you get the high level athletic performances. At the advanced HIIT level, you would increase your intensity and be doing twice the high-intensity to one period of rest, for ratio of 2 to 1. And at this level, you are doing very high intensity cardio workouts, such as squat jumps, burpees, or mountain climbers.

At the advanced level, you can keep your workout varied and more intense by combining exercises and making them more challenging. If you are doing squat jumps, for example, you can work on squatting as low as possible, and jumping as high as possible during the jump portion. This type of focus will allow you to fine-tune and increase your intensity levels at the advanced level.

Chapter 3

Combining Aerobic and Anaerobic Exercise

HIIT Training Program

One reason why HIIT workouts are so powerful is because aerobic and anaerobic exercises are combined and this provides massive health benefits. So what is the difference between the two?

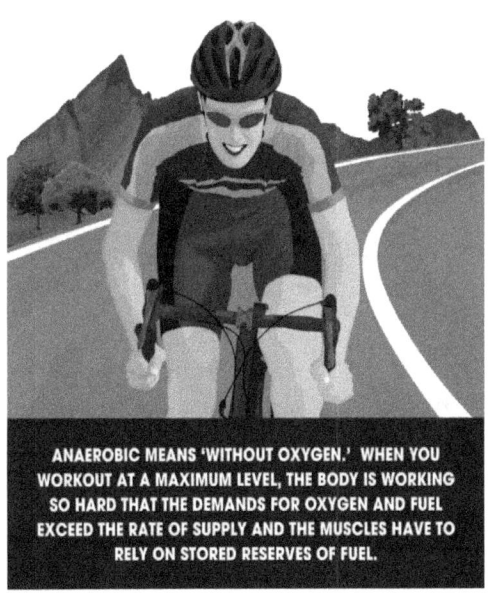

ANAEROBIC MEANS 'WITHOUT OXYGEN.' WHEN YOU WORKOUT AT A MAXIMUM LEVEL, THE BODY IS WORKING SO HARD THAT THE DEMANDS FOR OXYGEN AND FUEL EXCEED THE RATE OF SUPPLY AND THE MUSCLES HAVE TO RELY ON STORED RESERVES OF FUEL.

With anaerobic exercise, oxygen is not used as fuel as it is with aerobic exercise. Instead, glycogen is the fuel that is used to supply energy.

HIIT Training Program

Anaerobic exercise fatigues the body quickly and often within two hours of exercising, you will have depleted your glycogen and be incredibly fatigued. In fact, athletes tend to load up on carbohydrates to sustain energy when they are doing heavily anaerobic activities. Another thing is that anaerobic exercise was can lead to lactic acid buildup in the muscles, which leads to muscle soreness.

Anaerobic exercises include a variety of workouts that are done at maximum levels of intensity, such as weight lifting, kettle bells, sprints. These types of exercises have many benefits including:

- Increasing lean muscle mass, which makes burning calories faster and easier.

- Increasing the resting metabolism so you burn calories even when you're not working out.

- Increasing overall fitness levels by improving endurance.

HIIT Training Program

Anaerobic training is generally attained at around 75% of maximum heart rate. Anaerobic (HIIT) workouts are usually around 20-30 minutes of exertion.

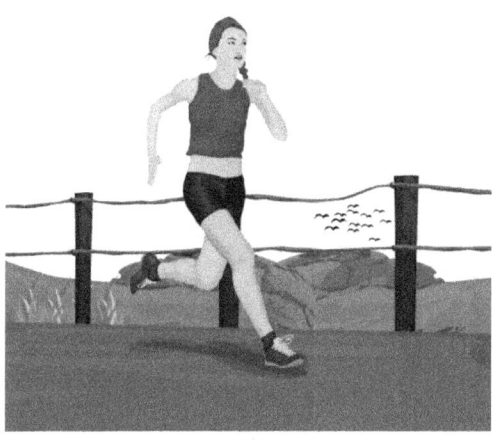

During aerobic exercise, your body relies a lot on oxygen to fuel energy, and you can actually experience tiredness and fatigue during your workout, if you don't have enough oxygen. The difference with aerobic exercises is that you can exercise for much more extended period of time than with anaerobic exercises. Also, with aerobic exercises you don't produce lactic acid as much which contributes to muscle soreness later.

HIIT Training Program

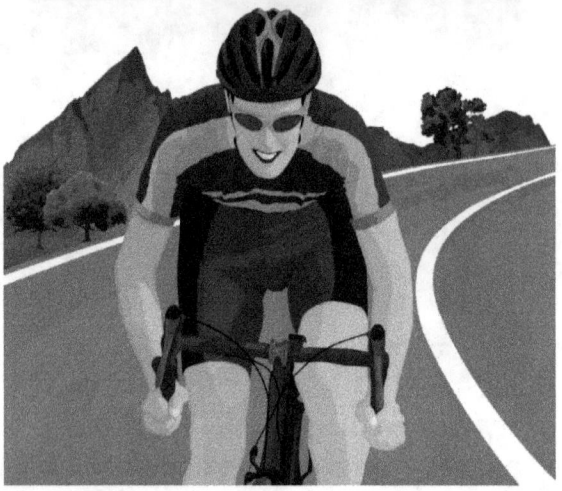

AEROBIC MEANS 'WITH OXYGEN.' DURING AEROBIC WORK THE BODY IS WORKING AT A LEVEL WHERE DEMANDS FOR OXYGEN AND FUEL CAN BE MET BY THE BODY'S INTAKE.

Aerobic exercise has a lot of benefits, including increasing your heart rate with exercises like running, rowing, and biking have a number of benefits including:

- Strengthening the lungs and the heart.

- Increasing endurance.

HIIT Training Program

- Releasing endorphins that prevent mood swings and depression.

- And many other benefits.

Both aerobic and anaerobic exercises have positives and negatives when done on their own. The magic happens when you combine these exercises in H IIT HIIT workouts. Your levels of fatigue will be much less, as you will not be depriving your body of oxygen (aerobic) or glycogen (anaerobic), b. Because you are doing short bursts. You do not suffer the drawbacks of longer workouts with fatigue or lactic acid buildup, but instead you will have the maximum health benefits.

Chapter 4

Increasing Energy with HIIT

HIIT Training Program

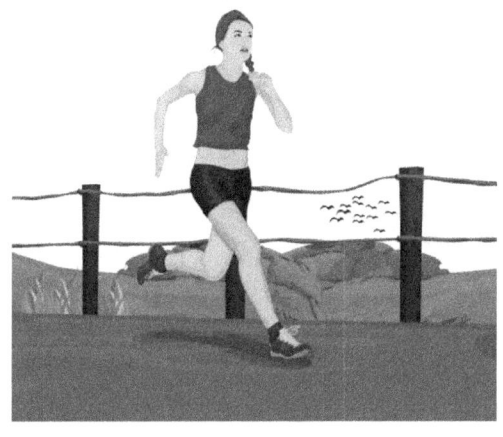

Start interval training with a 1:2 work to rest ratio. An example would be sprinting for 30 seconds and walking or slow jog to recover for one minute.

If you are comparing HIIT to a cardio only workout, you'll find that your overall energy levels will increase much more with HIIT. HIIT workouts are much shorter than the average cardio workout, so you don't expend all your energy exercising for an hour. Instead, the average workout tends to be about 15 minutes with a cool down.

Another reason energy levels are increased is because there is more oxygen being used by your body. Then there is with a regular cardio workout. Oxygen is the molecule which, when burned, helps your body. Take the carbs and fat and break it down to provide energy. When your body uses oxygen efficiently during exercise, use less of your energy and your body burns fat much more efficiently.

For example, when working at lower intensity, your body will become more efficient, so you can do the workout longer, but doesn't have as much power. However, higher intensity exercises like jumping rope kick in the anaerobic effect in your body requires a lot of oxygen in a short amount of time. This creates a very powerful metabolism, when you alternate those intense burst of exercises with intervals of lower intensity. This is why, with each HIIT session, your energy levels will be high, and you will also lose weight quicker and your fitness level will increase faster.

Chapter 5

Losing Weight with HIIT

HIIT Training Program

Choosing the HIIT approach over long cardio sessions is a more effective avenue to weight loss. With combining anaerobic activity in shorter workouts, your body will be building muscle and burning fat throughout the day.

The bottom line is that you can burn more calories with a 15 minute HIIT workout than a steady cardio workout. Studies have shown that after high-intensity training for six weeks, the participants received a number of benefits, including:

- A higher metabolic resting rate for up to 24 hours after their exercise session.
- A lower appetite.
- Higher levels of hormones that help fat loss.
- Improve sensitivity to insulin.

Most people today are short on time and energy. By working out the HIIT way you can increase your energy and reduce your workout time while increasing results.

Other Health Benefits of HIIT

Not only can you lose weight with H IIT, but research has shown that you can greatly improve your overall health and your fitness level. Here are some additional benefits:

- With many traditional exercise and diet programs. It can be difficult to keep muscle mass. When you're losing fat. HIIT lets you build and maintain muscle mass while you're burning calories.

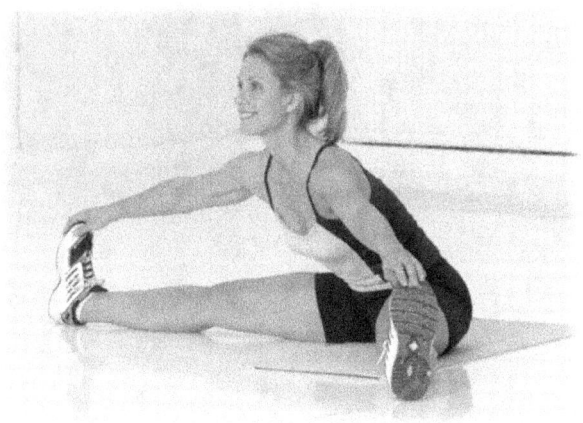

- Simulates HGH production. Human growth hormone production in our body tapers off as we get older. This hormone is important for slowing the aging process, and each HIIT workout increases HGH in some cases by up to 400%, so you'll feel younger.

- Improves blood sugar. Those with type II diabetes improved their blood sugar regulation after only working out two weeks with H IIT HIIT and doing three sessions weekly.

Chapter 6

Nutrition with HIIT

HIIT Training Program

To get the best results with H IIT, having a thought out nutrition plan will ensure that most benefits. The body needs to have enough glycogen to get through the high-intensity level intervals. In addition, hydration is incredibly important.

To prepare the body for the HIIT workout, a pre-workout meal is also essential. You should eat 2 to 3 hours before your workout and include fruit carbs and protein. Carbs will help you with the energy burst necessary for your workout to be most effective.

You do not need to eliminate any particular types of food, either. Using protein only, as some weight loss plans is not recommended, as it doesn't provide enough fuel. Of course you want to have protein, but during a workout, carbs are more beneficial. You can use carbs, very efficiently and effectively, so you don't want to cut them out of your diet.

Dairy has also been found to build muscle mass and decrease fat because of the calcium, vitamin D and protein. If you are lactose intolerant, there are a number of protein drinks available that you can have which could be considered a milk or a protein-based drink. Having something like this after your workout will help with your recovery.

Drinking plenty of water will help you flush out any toxins and HIIT requires lots of fluids. If you drink at least eight glasses of water a day, you will stay hydrated. Nutritional supplements are not necessary when you first get started with H IIT.

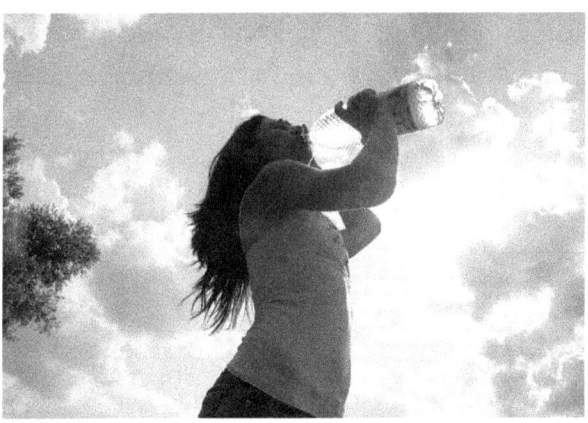

Fruit, vegetables, lean protein, carbohydrates and good fats are a strong diet for effective workouts. Because HIIT is burning carbs effectively, you can test how many carbs you'll need in your daily diet to see what works for you.

HIIT Training Program

Many higher-level athletes do use protein supplements to increase endurance during workouts that are high-intensity. These are usually consumed before you start working out. Another supplement that is popular, which helps minimize muscle fatigue, is beta alanine, an amino acid. In addition, after workout many athletes will have an additional protein supplement to provide energy and keep burning fat after the workout. However, this is not something you necessarily need to get started with the right way you can wait until you've built up some endurance and have adjusted your diet for the best benefits.

Chapter 7

Faster Workouts with HIIT

HIIT Training Program

Are you too busy for a long workout session? HIIT sessions are 15 minutes or less, and the results are even stronger than those achieved with long cardio workouts.

When you can't describe HIIT workouts is no sweat, the fact is that anyone can do intense energy in short bursts followed by a longer period of rest and recovery. This is one of the main reasons HIIT has exploded in popularity because of its core strengthening fat burning ability to scope the body.

The interval style training gets the heart rate up and really increases the metabolism so you are burning fat way after the workout is finished.

Adjusting HIIT Levels

As you progress through your workouts, you will find that you have to adjust your levels of intensity over time. You know you're ready to do this when you are not challenge in your workouts anymore.

When moving from the beginner to a more advanced level. Increase your overall workout

HIIT Training Program

time from 1 to 3 extra minutes. Another way you can do this is increase your higher-level intensity section, and decrease your recovery time. A common mistake made with this type of training is not putting in the recovery time. That recovery time is essential in order to get the benefits.

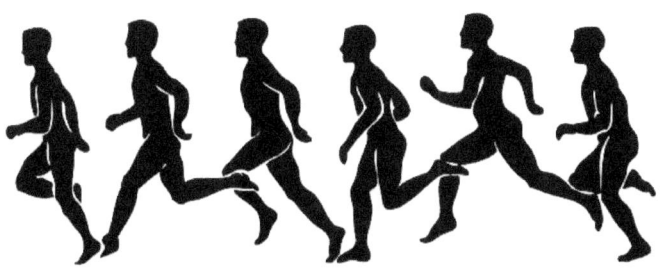

When you're first starting out, you would not be training every day, but perhaps a few times a week, so you can gradually build up your intensity. You can do other types of fitness in your additional workout sessions while you build up your workouts with HIIT.

Chapter 8

HIIT Workouts

HIIT Training Program

There are many different types of workouts and exercises you can do and turn them into an HIIT style workout here are some of the popular variations. Later in this book, I'll share some specific workouts with you.

- Gibala regimen-this is a great one to get started with. If you are not is used to exercising regularly. You start with a warm-up of three minutes, follow this with your intensity bursts of 60 seconds, and have a recovery period between each verse of about 20 seconds. Do this for 10 reps, and conclude with a five-minute cool down.

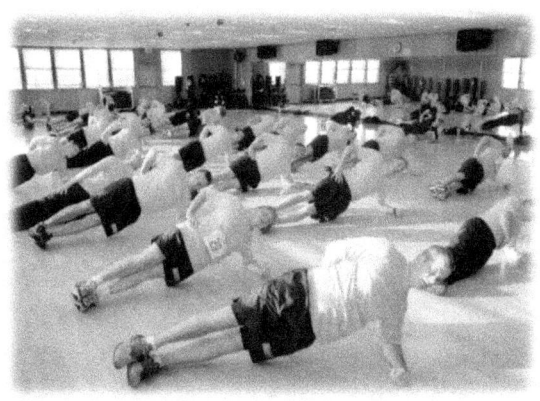

HIIT Training Program

- Tabata training-this cycle includes 20 seconds of intensity, with 10 seconds of recovery. The repetitions are eight times with this method.

- 10/20/30 Training-this is geared for runners and it is set up to run at a low speed for 30 seconds, amid speed for 20 seconds, and a Sprint for 10 seconds. This is repeated for five minutes with the recovery lasting for two minutes in between each interval. You can do this for 15 to 20 minutes and achieve great results.

- Little Method-this is an intermediate level workout. It starts with a warm-up of three minutes, 60 seconds of high intensity cycling, 75 seconds of slower cycling repeated for 12 sets total for time of 27 minutes.

- MetCon3-this is a free weight-based work out. You start with a warm-up, and then do free weight exercises, one set each done right after the other. The recovery is two minutes between each session and the sessions are repeated twice, and concluded with a cool down.

- Zumba-believe it or not, the Zumba is a HIIT work out. This popular dance workout starts gradually in becomes very intense, with short recovery periods between the intensity level training. You can workout at home with the DVD, or even join a class.

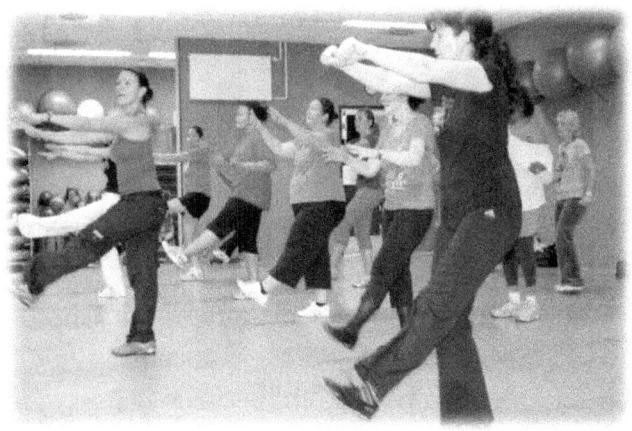

With HIIT, you can do many types of different exercises, putting the spin on it means that you are structuring it where you're doing short bursts of energy with shorter rest a recovery periods in between. This is great because it means you can try different exercises and not get bored doing the same thing.

One of the most important aspects of using HIIT is hitting the right HIIT ratio between high intensity activity and active resting periods. According to studies, the best ratio of work to rest is around 2:1. To simplify it, you should work intensely for two minutes and rest for one. While HIIT might be tough, finding the optimal ratio is actually pretty easy.

The problem with the above ratio is that it's best for athletes, but it may not suit someone who is just starting a HIIT routine, or someone who hasn't exercised in years. Your specific ratio should give you adequate time to recover after the intense side of your routine. If you need a few minutes, then it's fine. The point is that you get enough rest to perform at your best.

Another thing to consider is reps and weather. For example, working outdoors during the summer will make it harder to recover when compared to mild seasons, such as early fall or spring.

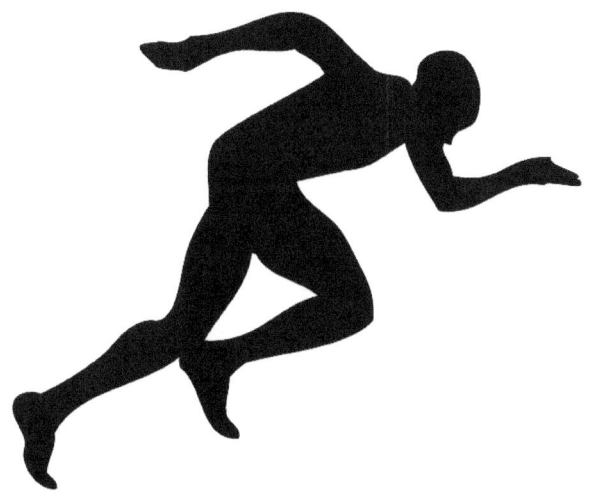

You'll also need to think about the specific type of exercise you're doing. Sprinting takes much more energy and effort than swimming for the exact same time ratio, so you might need to rest longer.

Following the Tabata HIIT routine burns a massive number of calories, but the routine might be too intense for beginners. Here's a typically ratio using two common exercise techniques: burpees and squat jumps:

HIIT Training Program

- Start with a five minute warm up.

- Follow the scientific ratio of 2:1, or 30 seconds of intense activity followed by 15 seconds of rest.

- Start with burpees. This starts from a plank or push up position, and takes you to standing, which primarily uses buttocks and leg muscles, and the core is targeted as well.

- Next, do squat jumps. You'll be focusing on many of the main leg muscles, including the thighs, calves and buttocks. Just like with burpees, the core is also activated.

- Alternate between the two moves for four minutes. Then, take a rest for two minutes before starting again.

Tabata is a favorite among HIIT enthusiasts, and it's great for burning calories in a very brief amount of time. Not only that, but it's typically not as exhausting as longer HIIT routines.

HIIT Training Program

Though the routine is fairly simple, it can be brutal the first few times. Start slowly and work your way to a lower resting ratio. There's no reason to kill yourself, just rest as long as you need to. You'll quickly see results with this routine.

Chapter 9

What You Can Expect With HIIT

HIIT Training Program

Now that you have the basics of HIIT, I'm sure you're ready to get started. Because you'll start seeing results in a short amount of time, it is easy to stay motivated because you will be able to work out for shorter durations and see better results. In the next section, I'll share with you some detailed HIIT workouts so you can get started and then once you gotten comfortable, you can then change up your routine.

You'll start to see significant results. After eight weeks of HIIT training here are some of the typical results from a workout regimen of eight weeks:

- Metabolism working better-studies have shown that those who did HIIT with the stationary bike burned more calories in the next 24 hours after the workout and those who cycled at a more moderate pace for a longer period of time.

- Burning more fat HIIT workout increases fat burning by about 50%. It also increases muscle proteins that moves that to be used for fuel in the cells.

HIIT Training Program

- 2% loss of body fat-studies of shown that people who followed this regimen for eight weeks loss of body fat percentage of 2% compared to those who did the regular exercise workout. In fact, the regular exercisers lost, nobody fat, and similar results have been seen from other studies.

Not only will you get these health benefits. If you stick to your HIIT regimen, but you'll have more energy and feel more confident, because you'll see results faster, without putting in the long hours at the gym. While the actual workouts themselves are challenging, you'll be having fun and enjoying the results that you'll come to relish that challenge over time.

Give HIIT a try and commit to eight weeks of workouts. Start with a few days a week, and you can increase your workout intensity, and add an extra day or two after your level of fitness increases.

Chapter 10

HITT Workouts to Get Started With

HIIT Training Program

The truth is that no equipment is needed to perform the HIIT routine, but it can still be used if you have access to and enjoy said equipment. As long as you perform the proper intervals of intense activity and recover, then you'll be following the HIIT philosophy while making an exceptional difference to your workout results.

However, just remember that equipment isn't really needed. Most people who do HIIT prefer to just use their body because machines can be boring, and they often only do aerobic or anaerobic work, whereas HIIT does both at once and in less time. You'll also burn calories and build more muscle by using HIIT with your machines.

If you do want to use equipment, then these are the best machines to use:

- Treadmill: Bored with your normal treadmill stroll or run? HIIT will reinvigorate your machine so that you like it again. Just follow the principles of doing several minutes of sprinting on an incline followed by a slow stroll to get your wind back.

HIIT Training Program

- Rowing Machine: Add HIIT to your rowing machine by rowing as quickly as possible for a specific number of miles, and then take a good rest. It's a powerful workout that will make your lungs burn.

- Free Weights: If you don't know already, weight lifting has some serious cardio benefits, and it transforms your body in a fat-burning machine. Just do some fast lifting (with the right amount of weight, of course), and you'll be surprised by how winded you are. Not only that, but you're toning both your muscles and lungs at the same time.

- Elliptical: Unlike a treadmill, ellipticals allow you to go as fast as you want. Push the incline up as far as possible and sprint for several minutes before taking a well-deserved rest. You'll be amazed at how hard, and beneficial, your elliptical becomes.

- Kettlebells: Kettlebells are like free weights on steroids. Not only do they provide a

better aerobic experience, but they also
work all of your muscles at once for overall
toning and muscle building. You'll also be
surprised by just how effective kettlebells
can be.

As you can see, HIIT works both with and without
machines, which allows you to do it anywhere and
with nearly anything. You'll be seeing your old
equipment in a whole new way after transforming
them with the HIIT philosophy. Not only that, but
you'll be getting even better results than with your
old, slow routine.

Specific HIIT Workouts

1. *12 Minute HIIT Weight or Kettlebell routine*
This is a great 12 minute workout; you can do with
dumbbells and/or kettle bells. You'll also want to
start off with 2-3 minutes of warm-up, like jogging.

HIIT Training Program

12 Minute HIIT Kettlebell or Weight Routine

Equipment
- interval timer or clock with second hand
- box for box jumps
- kettlebell
- sandbag, weighted vest, or dumbbells

Sets. For the intervals in this workout, you'll be performing high intensity exercises for 30 seconds with 10 minute rest periods in between. Once you've completed all the intervals once, you'll repeat them for a total of 3 cycles.

Interval 1 – Box Jumps – Do as many box jumps as you can for 30 seconds and then rest for 10 seconds.

Interval 2 – Kettlebell swings – Stand with wide legs and hold your kettlebell with both hands. Start with the kettlebell between your legs and swing it directly overhead. Return to the starting position. Repeat as many times as you can for 30 seconds. Rest for 10 seconds.

Interval 3 – Elevated pushups – Get in a pushup position with your feet elevated on your box so that they're elevated above your shoulders. Perform as many full pushups as you can for 30 seconds. Rest for 10 seconds.

Interval 4 – Side lunges – Perform lunges alternating on your left and right sides for 30 seconds. Rest for 10 seconds.

Interval 5 – Sit-ups – Perform as many full sit-ups as you can for 30 seconds. Rest for 10 seconds.

2. Cycling HIIT routine for beginners

Cycling is great for HIIT training. You can do it on a stationary bike or a road bike. Basically, you would have a high intensity level of cycling from

HIIT Training Program

anywhere to 30 to 90 seconds. Follow this with a shorter recovery time, and then you can repeat the number of cycles as often as you want for complete workout.

Here is a routine you can do on a stationary bike.

Beginner Cycling HIIT Routine

Equipment
- Road or stationary bike

5 minute warm up. This is a time for you to allow your muscles and joints to warm up preventing injury. At this point cycle with low-medium resistance on your bike and don't worry about speed – use a low level of energy.

Intervals. As a beginner, keep the resistance low on your bike until you're more familiar with this routine. The interval suggestions below may be very challenging. If you can't complete all of them, do the best you can and increase your intervals a little at a time.

A high intensity interval is a time when you're pedaling as fast as you can with as much energy as you have. The actual speed will vary depending on your current level of fitness. These are the recommended intervals:

- 30 seconds high intensity, 2 minutes low intensity (repeat 5 times)
- 40 seconds high intensity, 2 minutes low intensity (repeat 5 times)
- 30 seconds high intensity, 1 minute low intensity (repeat 5 times)

5 Minute Cool Down. A cool down allows you to get your heart rate back to normal and allows your muscles to have some recovery time as well. Cycle with low energy for five minutes.

Stretch. Any workout should be followed by a stretching routine. For cycling your lower body is most engaged. It's important so stretch your calves, quads, hamstrings, glutes, and don't forget about your ankles and feet.

HIIT Training Program

3. HIIT Running Routine For Beginners

All you need for running is a pair of good shoes. Running lends itself well to HIIT because you can focus on increasing your intensity levels over time without having to run long distances. The best way to get started with this routine is to run on a track first, overtime you can then run on trails or other types of terrain.

HIIT Training Program

Running Track HIIT Routine for Beginners

Equipment
- Indoor or outdoor track

High Intensity Intervals: Once you've warmed up, you'll begin adding high intensity intervals.

Beginner Intervals: Sprint for 30 seconds, then walk or jog for 5 minutes (repeat 5 times)

Intermediate to Advanced Intervals: This entire routine will take approximately 30 minutes. If this routine seems easy for you, you can vary the cycle to add more intervals.

For example:

- Sprint for 30 seconds, then jog for 2 minutes at an easy pace (repeat 5 times)
- Sprint for 30 seconds, then jog for 3 minutes at an easy pace (repeat 5 times)
- Sprint for 30 seconds, then jog for 3 minutes at an easy pace (repeat 5 times)

You can add to the workout by repeating the cycles more than 5 times or by decreasing the recovery time in between intervals. However, you should always allow for 90 second recoveries between intervals.

HIIT Training Program

4. Killer Ab Workout

You can target and strengthen your core with this fantastic workout. You just need a floor mat, and an interval timer or stopwatch for this workout.

HIIT Routine for Killer Abs

Equipment
- None

Intervals. Each of these intervals needs to be performed for 45 seconds with as much speed and energy as you can give. Following the speed interval, rest for 15 seconds.

Interval 1 – Bicycle Crunches. Lie on your back without letting your feet touch the ground. Place your hands at the side of your head with bent elbows. Bring your right knee to your chest while twisting your left elbow to touch your knee (keeping your left leg parallel to your body without touching the floor). Then switch legs and twist the other direction. Repeat this for 45 seconds and then rest for 15 seconds.

Interval 2 – Jumping Jacks. Perform jumping jacks as fast as you can for 45 seconds and then rest for 15 seconds.

Interval 3 – Flutter Kicks. Lie on your back and place your hands to the side of your head or place them below your buttocks. Lift your right leg into the air while keeping your left leg down, but not touching the floor. Lower your right leg and lift your left leg. Repeat this for 45 seconds. Rest for 15 seconds.

Interval 4 – Squat Knee Lift Combo. Stand with your feet hip width apart and your arms at your sides. Lower your body into a squat and raise your arms in front of you. Stand up from the squat and raise your right knee. Return to a stand and repeat the squat then raise your left knee. Repeat this combination for 45 seconds and rest for 15 seconds.

Interval 5 – Mountain Climbers. Get into a plank position on the floor with your arms straight in front of you and your back straight. Keep your legs shoulder width apart. Bring your right knee toward your chest. Straighten your right knee while bringing in your left knee. Repeat for 45 seconds and rest for 15.

---

5. *Tabata Training HIIT Style*

Tabata training was created by Dr. Isumi Tabata 'who did a number of studies showing how effective it can be. While the core training method is only 4 minutes of exercise, a warm-up and cool down does need to be included and the exercised duration can be extended.

Here is a standard routine you can modify for a daily practice.

HIIT Training Program

Tabata HIIT Routine

Equipment
*   None

Warm Up. Start by walking or jogging in place for five minutes. You just want to get enough movement to warm up your muscles and loosen your joints.

Intervals. With Tabata you'll choose four exercises to perform. In this example routine you'll be performing:

*   jumping jacks
*   high knees
*   squats
*   pushups

Begin by doing jumping jacks as fast as you can for 20 seconds. Then you'll rest for 10 seconds. Then you'll move on to high knees for 20 seconds and rest for 10 seconds. Continue on with squats and pushups in the same manner.

After you've gone through all four exercises , repeat the cycle one more time.

Cool Down. Following the 4 minutes of HIIT you'll need to cool down. You can walk or jog anywhere from 5-10 minutes. In Tabata research studies, the cool down was performed for the entire 10 minutes.

Chapter 11

Conclusion

HIIT Training Program

With a little training and practice, you can quickly achieve massive results from HIIT. Don't neglect this powerful type of training that can be adapted to a large variety of workouts.

Let's stay in touch! You can pick up a free guide to Tabata training and some additional tips to keep you on track, here:

http://ebooknicheclub.com/FastFitness/index.html

Recommended Resources

HIIT Training Program

Websites/Blog Posts

http://blog.fitbug.com/hiit-craze-good-bad-ugly-high-intensity-interval-training/

http://well.blogs.nytimes.com/2014/02/26/how-to-get-fit-in-a-few-minutes-a-week/?_php=true&_type=blogs&_r=0

http://www.workingmother.com/blogs/mojo-coach/high-intensity-interval-training-huge-fitness-hit-busy-moms

http://www.chicagonow.com/get-fit-chicago/2014/01/a-fat-burning-high-intensity-interval-training-workout-anyone-can-do/

http://8fit.com/blog/hiit/

http://bakingdietitian.weebly.com/blog/hiit-high-intensity-interval-training-workouts

http://www.fitness19.com/trending-now-high-intensity-interval-training-in-2014/

https://www.vidafitnessblog.com/maximizing-cardio-workouts-benefits-high-intensity-interval-training/

http://www.clubsatcrp.com/fitness-blog/high-intensity-interval-training/

HIIT Training Program

http://www.myprotein.com/thezone/mens/lose-weight-fast-high-intensity-interval-training/

Videos

http://youtu.be/8s8SY_2Lhrk

http://youtu.be/k3kiQ4lhD4g

http://youtu.be/xKVZp-ZLDKE

http://youtu.be/_6sbiVRYsGE

http://youtu.be/NbFTEKLK92U

http://youtu.be/VOHikFY0nBY

http://youtu.be/04-VoVzOiSg

http://youtu.be/bDAG3B-XiOo

http://youtu.be/D0rtkcbSUHM

http://youtu.be/SwJUR9mHL1Y